I0414046

Homemade Lotions
40 Best Organic Lotion Recipes

Table of content

Introduction

There you are, at the store once more, looking to find a lotion that is going to work on your sensitive skin and not slather you with chemicals you don't want to put on your body.

If you have ever done any research on the way your skin absorbs, you know that everything you rub into your skin is going to end up inside you, and you know you have to be careful about the things you decide to do that with.

Whether you are worried about illness, toxic buildup, or you are just on the health conscious side, you know that you have to be careful about what you put in your body, or on your body for that matter, and lotions can be one of the most harmful things you could buy if you aren't careful!

Thankfully, you can now avoid all of that and make your own lotions. You can create the blend that is right for you, and you can mix and match to make it just what you want it to be, without worry that you are putting things on your skin that you shouldn't be.

Use organic ingredients, have fun while you do it, and make the most out of the things you put on your skin, and you are going to get the results you are after in a matter of hours. Try out any of these lotions just once, and you will be hooked for life.

So if you are ready to step out of the toxins that they put in the lotions today, and jump into the organic and healthy life, you have come to the right place. Let this book be your guide in the realm of lotion making, and put your mind at ease as you pamper yourself pretty.

Relax, you deserve this.

Chapter 1 – Basic Lotions For Everyone

Mom's Favorite Lotion

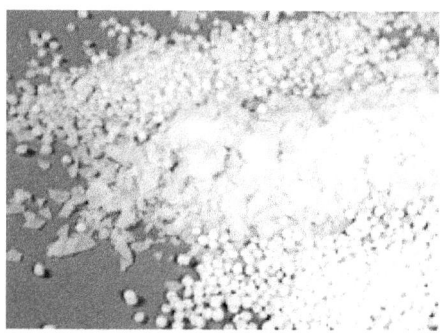

10 drops rose oil

10 drops lavender

1/8 cup shea butter

1/8 cup shredded mango butter

1/8 cup beeswax cubes

¼ cup coconut oil

3 teaspoons sweet almond oil

Directions:

Turn a saucepan onto medium low heat on your stove. Carefully scoop in the beeswax and stir until melted, then add in the shea butter and mango butter. Stir until these are melted as well.

Once you have a completely smooth blend, add in your coconut oil and almond oil, then the drops of essential oils.

Again, blend with a wooden spoon until completely smooth and carefully pour into airtight glass jars for storage.

When you are ready to use, simply scoop a small section out with your fingers (it will be firm) and let soften, then massage into your skin, and that's it!

Fun in the Fields

10 drops rosewood

10 drops lilac

4 drops wheatgrass

1/8 cup shea butter

1/8 cup shredded mango butter

1/8 cup beeswax cubes

¼ cup coconut oil

3 teaspoons sweet almond oil

Directions:

Turn a saucepan onto medium low heat on your stove. Carefully scoop in the beeswax and stir until melted, then add in the shea butter and mango butter. Stir until these are melted as well.

Once you have a completely smooth blend, add in your coconut oil and almond oil, then the drops of essential oils.

Again, blend with a wooden spoon until completely smooth and carefully pour into airtight glass jars for storage.

When you are ready to use, simply scoop a small section out with your fingers (it will be firm) and let soften, then massage into your skin, and that's it!

Grandma's Best Lotion

10 drops cupcake aroma therapy oil

5 drops clean linen oil

5 drops rosemary oil

1/8 cup shea butter

1/8 cup shredded mango butter

1/8 cup beeswax cubes

¼ cup coconut oil

3 teaspoons sweet almond oil

Directions:

Turn a saucepan onto medium low heat on your stove. Carefully scoop in the beeswax and stir until melted, then add in the shea butter and mango butter. Stir until these are melted as well.

Once you have a completely smooth blend, add in your coconut oil and almond oil, then the drops of essential oils.

Again, blend with a wooden spoon until completely smooth and carefully pour into airtight glass jars for storage.

When you are ready to use, simply scoop a small section out with your fingers (it will be firm) and let soften, then massage into your skin, and that's it!

Utterly Smooth Hands

10 drops geranium oil

10 drops sandalwood

10 drops tea tree oil

1/8 cup shea butter

1/8 cup shredded mango butter

1/8 cup beeswax cubes

¼ cup coconut oil

3 teaspoons sweet almond oil

Directions:

Turn a saucepan onto medium low heat on your stove. Carefully scoop in the beeswax and stir until melted, then add in the shea butter and mango butter. Stir until these are melted as well.

Once you have a completely smooth blend, add in your coconut oil and almond oil, then the drops of essential oils.

Again, blend with a wooden spoon until completely smooth and carefully pour into airtight glass jars for storage.

When you are ready to use, simply scoop a small section out with your fingers (it will be firm) and let soften, then massage into your skin, and that's it!

The Winner

10 drops frankincense oil

5 drops lavender oil

5 drops myrrh oil

1/8 cup shea butter

1/8 cup shredded mango butter

1/8 cup beeswax cubes

¼ cup coconut oil

3 teaspoons sweet almond oil

Directions:

Turn a saucepan onto medium low heat on your stove. Carefully scoop in the beeswax and stir until melted, then add in the shea butter and mango butter. Stir until these are melted as well.

Once you have a completely smooth blend, add in your coconut oil and almond oil, then the drops of essential oils.

Again, blend with a wooden spoon until completely smooth and carefully pour into airtight glass jars for storage.

When you are ready to use, simply scoop a small section out with your fingers (it will be firm) and let soften, then massage into your skin, and that's it!

Do What You Want

10 drops orange oil

10 drops sweet orange oil

5 drops citrus oil

1/8 cup shea butter

1/8 cup shredded mango butter

1/8 cup beeswax cubes

¼ cup coconut oil

3 teaspoons sweet almond oil

Directions:

Turn a saucepan onto medium low heat on your stove. Carefully scoop in the beeswax and stir until melted, then add in the shea butter and mango butter. Stir until these are melted as well.

Once you have a completely smooth blend, add in your coconut oil and almond oil, then the drops of essential oils.

Again, blend with a wooden spoon until completely smooth and carefully pour into airtight glass jars for storage.

When you are ready to use, simply scoop a small section out with your fingers (it will be firm) and let soften, then massage into your skin, and that's it!

Everyone's Gone Green Lotion

10 drops tea tree oil

5 drops wheatgrass oil

1 tablespoon green tea

1/8 cup shea butter

1/8 cup shredded mango butter

1/8 cup beeswax cubes

¼ cup coconut oil

3 teaspoons sweet almond oil

Directions:

Turn a saucepan onto medium low heat on your stove. Carefully scoop in the beeswax and stir until melted, then add in the shea butter and mango butter. Stir until these are melted as well.

Once you have a completely smooth blend, add in your coconut oil and almond oil, then the drops of essential oils.

Again, blend with a wooden spoon until completely smooth and carefully pour into airtight glass jars for storage.

When you are ready to use, simply scoop a small section out with your fingers (it will be firm) and let soften, then massage into your skin, and that's it!

Just What You Needed

10 drops spearmint oil

10 drops peppermint oil

10 drops lavender oil

1/8 cup shea butter

1/8 cup shredded mango butter

1/8 cup beeswax cubes

¼ cup coconut oil

3 teaspoons sweet almond oil

Directions:

Turn a saucepan onto medium low heat on your stove. Carefully scoop in the beeswax and stir until melted, then add in the shea butter and mango butter. Stir until these are melted as well.

Once you have a completely smooth blend, add in your coconut oil and almond oil, then the drops of essential oils.

Again, blend with a wooden spoon until completely smooth and carefully pour into airtight glass jars for storage.

When you are ready to use, simply scoop a small section out with your fingers (it will be firm) and let soften, then massage into your skin, and that's it!

Chapter 2 – Lots of Love Lotions

The Heart Throb Lotion

10 drops licorice aroma therapy oil

5 drops lavender oil

5 drops orange oil

1/8 cup shea butter

1/8 cup shredded mango butter

1/8 cup beeswax cubes

¼ cup coconut oil

3 teaspoons sweet almond oil

Directions:

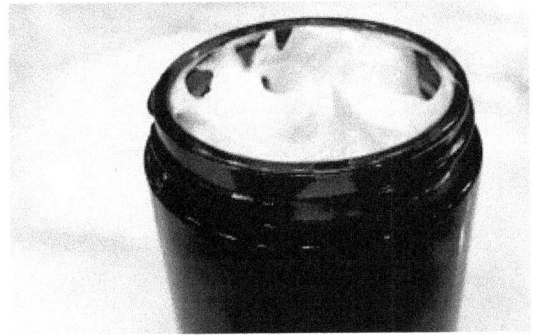

Turn a saucepan onto medium low heat on your stove. Carefully scoop in the beeswax and stir until melted, then add in the shea butter and mango butter. Stir until these are melted as well.

Once you have a completely smooth blend, add in your coconut oil and almond oil, then the drops of essential oils.

Again, blend with a wooden spoon until completely smooth and carefully pour into airtight glass jars for storage.

When you are ready to use, simply scoop a small section out with your fingers (it will be firm) and let soften, then massage into your skin, and that's it!

Kiss of Love Lotion

10 drops myrrh oil

12 drops bubblegum aromatherapy oil

1/8 cup shea butter

1/8 cup shredded mango butter

1/8 cup beeswax cubes

¼ cup coconut oil

3 teaspoons sweet almond oil

Directions:

Turn a saucepan onto medium low heat on your stove. Carefully scoop in the beeswax and stir until melted, then add in the shea butter and mango butter. Stir until these are melted as well.

Once you have a completely smooth blend, add in your coconut oil and almond oil, then the drops of essential oils.

Again, blend with a wooden spoon until completely smooth and carefully pour into airtight glass jars for storage.

When you are ready to use, simply scoop a small section out with your fingers (it will be firm) and let soften, then massage into your skin, and that's it!

X's And O's

10 drops sweet orange oil

5 drops vanilla essential oil

1/8 cup shea butter

1/8 cup shredded mango butter

1/8 cup beeswax cubes

¼ cup coconut oil

3 teaspoons sweet almond oil

Directions:

Turn a saucepan onto medium low heat on your stove. Carefully scoop in the beeswax and stir until melted, then add in the shea butter and mango butter. Stir until these are melted as well.

Once you have a completely smooth blend, add in your coconut oil and almond oil, then the drops of essential oils.

Again, blend with a wooden spoon until completely smooth and carefully pour into airtight glass jars for storage.

When you are ready to use, simply scoop a small section out with your fingers (it will be firm) and let soften, then massage into your skin, and that's it!

From Mine To Yours

10 drops peppermint oil

10 drops bubblegum aromatherapy oil

5 drops rose oil

1/8 cup shea butter

1/8 cup shredded mango butter

1/8 cup beeswax cubes

¼ cup coconut oil

3 teaspoons sweet almond oil

Directions:

Turn a saucepan onto medium low heat on your stove. Carefully scoop in the beeswax and stir until melted, then add in the shea butter and mango butter. Stir until these are melted as well.

Once you have a completely smooth blend, add in your coconut oil and almond oil, then the drops of essential oils.

Again, blend with a wooden spoon until completely smooth and carefully pour into airtight glass jars for storage.

When you are ready to use, simply scoop a small section out with your fingers (it will be firm) and let soften, then massage into your skin, and that's it!

Can You Feel the Love?

10 drops grapefruit oil

5 drops white musk aromatherapy oil

4 drops bergamot

1/8 cup shea butter

1/8 cup shredded mango butter

1/8 cup beeswax cubes

¼ cup coconut oil

3 teaspoons sweet almond oil

Directions:

Turn a saucepan onto medium low heat on your stove. Carefully scoop in the beeswax and stir until melted, then add in the shea butter and mango butter. Stir until these are melted as well.

Once you have a completely smooth blend, add in your coconut oil and almond oil, then the drops of essential oils.

Again, blend with a wooden spoon until completely smooth and carefully pour into airtight glass jars for storage.

When you are ready to use, simply scoop a small section out with your fingers (it will be firm) and let soften, then massage into your skin, and that's it!

His and Hers

8 drops rosemary

8 drops rosewood

8 drops rose

10 drops patchouli

1/8 cup shea butter

1/8 cup shredded mango butter

1/8 cup beeswax cubes

¼ cup coconut oil

3 teaspoons sweet almond oil

Directions:

Turn a saucepan onto medium low heat on your stove. Carefully scoop in the beeswax and stir until melted, then add in the shea butter and mango butter. Stir until these are melted as well.

Once you have a completely smooth blend, add in your coconut oil and almond oil, then the drops of essential oils.

Again, blend with a wooden spoon until completely smooth and carefully pour into airtight glass jars for storage.

When you are ready to use, simply scoop a small section out with your fingers (it will be firm) and let soften, then massage into your skin, and that's it!

Two's for Two

12 drops patchouli

10 drops geranium

10 drops lavender

10 drops rose oil

1/8 cup shea butter

1/8 cup shredded mango butter

1/8 cup beeswax cubes

¼ cup coconut oil

3 teaspoons sweet almond oil

Directions:

Turn a saucepan onto medium low heat on your stove. Carefully scoop in the beeswax and stir until melted, then add in the shea butter and mango butter. Stir until these are melted as well.

Once you have a completely smooth blend, add in your coconut oil and almond oil, then the drops of essential oils.

Again, blend with a wooden spoon until completely smooth and carefully pour into airtight glass jars for storage.

When you are ready to use, simply scoop a small section out with your fingers (it will be firm) and let soften, then massage into your skin, and that's it!

The Wingman Lotion

8 drops white musk aromatherapy oil

8 drops vanilla oil

5 drops myrrh

1/8 cup shea butter

1/8 cup shredded mango butter

1/8 cup beeswax cubes

¼ cup coconut oil

3 teaspoons sweet almond oil

Directions:

Turn a saucepan onto medium low heat on your stove. Carefully scoop in the beeswax and stir until melted, then add in the shea butter and mango butter. Stir until these are melted as well.

Once you have a completely smooth blend, add in your coconut oil and almond oil, then the drops of essential oils.

Again, blend with a wooden spoon until completely smooth and carefully pour into airtight glass jars for storage.

When you are ready to use, simply scoop a small section out with your fingers (it will be firm) and let soften, then massage into your skin, and that's it!

Chapter 3 – A Little Here A Little There

The Cat's Eye Lotion

10 drops tiger lily oil

8 drops sandalwood

1/8 cup shea butter

1/8 cup shredded mango butter

1/8 cup beeswax cubes

¼ cup coconut oil

3 teaspoons sweet almond oil

Directions:

Turn a saucepan onto medium low heat on your stove. Carefully scoop in the beeswax and stir until melted, then add in the shea butter and mango butter. Stir until these are melted as well.

Once you have a completely smooth blend, add in your coconut oil and almond oil, then the drops of essential oils.

Again, blend with a wooden spoon until completely smooth and carefully pour into airtight glass jars for storage.

When you are ready to use, simply scoop a small section out with your fingers (it will be firm) and let soften, then massage into your skin, and that's it!

Kiss of the Sun

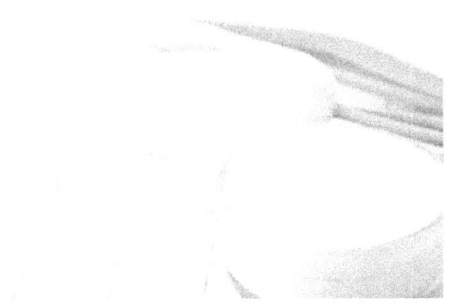

10 drops cedar

12 drops grapefruit

10 drops blood orange

1/8 cup shea butter

1/8 cup shredded mango butter

1/8 cup beeswax cubes

¼ cup coconut oil

3 teaspoons sweet almond oil

Directions:

Turn a saucepan onto medium low heat on your stove. Carefully scoop in the beeswax and stir until melted, then add in the shea butter and mango butter. Stir until these are melted as well.

Once you have a completely smooth blend, add in your coconut oil and almond oil, then the drops of essential oils.

Again, blend with a wooden spoon until completely smooth and carefully pour into airtight glass jars for storage.

When you are ready to use, simply scoop a small section out with your fingers (it will be firm) and let soften, then massage into your skin, and that's it!

Citrus Song Lotion

10 drops lemon

10 drops lime

10 drops orange

1/8 cup shea butter

1/8 cup shredded mango butter

1/8 cup beeswax cubes

¼ cup coconut oil

3 teaspoons sweet almond oil

Directions:

Turn a saucepan onto medium low heat on your stove. Carefully scoop in the beeswax and stir until melted, then add in the shea butter and mango butter. Stir until these are melted as well.

Once you have a completely smooth blend, add in your coconut oil and almond oil, then the drops of essential oils.

Again, blend with a wooden spoon until completely smooth and carefully pour into airtight glass jars for storage.

When you are ready to use, simply scoop a small section out with your fingers (it will be firm) and let soften, then massage into your skin, and that's it!

Fresh Air Blast

12 drops peppermint

10 drops eucalyptus

8 drops tea tree

1/8 cup shea butter

1/8 cup shredded mango butter

1/8 cup beeswax cubes

¼ cup coconut oil

3 teaspoons sweet almond oil

Directions:

Turn a saucepan onto medium low heat on your stove. Carefully scoop in the beeswax and stir until melted, then add in the shea butter and mango butter. Stir until these are melted as well.

Once you have a completely smooth blend, add in your coconut oil and almond oil, then the drops of essential oils.

Again, blend with a wooden spoon until completely smooth and carefully pour into airtight glass jars for storage.

When you are ready to use, simply scoop a small section out with your fingers (it will be firm) and let soften, then massage into your skin, and that's it!

Smooth and Silky Love

10 drops grapefruit

10 drops lilac

10 drops myrrh

8 drops sunflower oil

1/8 cup shea butter

1/8 cup shredded mango butter

1/8 cup beeswax cubes

¼ cup coconut oil

3 teaspoons sweet almond oil

Directions:

Turn a saucepan onto medium low heat on your stove. Carefully scoop in the beeswax and stir until melted, then add in the shea butter and mango butter. Stir until these are melted as well.

Once you have a completely smooth blend, add in your coconut oil and almond oil, then the drops of essential oils.

Again, blend with a wooden spoon until completely smooth and carefully pour into airtight glass jars for storage.

When you are ready to use, simply scoop a small section out with your fingers (it will be firm) and let soften, then massage into your skin, and that's it!

Walking on Air

10 drops cinnamon

8 drops lemon oil

8 drops lemongrass

1/8 cup shea butter

1/8 cup shredded mango butter

1/8 cup beeswax cubes

¼ cup coconut oil

3 teaspoons sweet almond oil

Directions:

Turn a saucepan onto medium low heat on your stove. Carefully scoop in the beeswax and stir until melted, then add in the shea butter and mango butter. Stir until these are melted as well.

Once you have a completely smooth blend, add in your coconut oil and almond oil, then the drops of essential oils.

Again, blend with a wooden spoon until completely smooth and carefully pour into airtight glass jars for storage.

When you are ready to use, simply scoop a small section out with your fingers (it will be firm) and let soften, then massage into your skin, and that's it!

Breezy Balm

10 drops grapefruit

8 drops pineapple aromatherapy oil

8 drops lemon

1/8 cup shea butter

1/8 cup shredded mango butter

1/8 cup beeswax cubes

¼ cup coconut oil

3 teaspoons sweet almond oil

Directions:

Turn a saucepan onto medium low heat on your stove. Carefully scoop in the beeswax and stir until melted, then add in the shea butter and mango butter. Stir until these are melted as well.

Once you have a completely smooth blend, add in your coconut oil and almond oil, then the drops of essential oils.

Again, blend with a wooden spoon until completely smooth and carefully pour into airtight glass jars for storage.

When you are ready to use, simply scoop a small section out with your fingers (it will be firm) and let soften, then massage into your skin, and that's it!

Sweets to the Sweet

10 drops cotton candy aromatherapy oil

5 drops cinnamon

5 drops vanilla oil

1/8 cup shea butter

1/8 cup shredded mango butter

1/8 cup beeswax cubes

¼ cup coconut oil

3 teaspoons sweet almond oil

Directions:

Turn a saucepan onto medium low heat on your stove. Carefully scoop in the beeswax and stir until melted, then add in the shea butter and mango butter. Stir until these are melted as well.

Once you have a completely smooth blend, add in your coconut oil and almond oil, then the drops of essential oils.

Again, blend with a wooden spoon until completely smooth and carefully pour into airtight glass jars for storage.

When you are ready to use, simply scoop a small section out with your fingers (it will be firm) and let soften, then massage into your skin, and that's it!

Chapter 4 – Holidays Every Day Lotions

Christmas in August

12 drops peppermint

12 drops cinnamon

12 drops ginger

1/8 cup shea butter

1/8 cup shredded mango butter

1/8 cup beeswax cubes

¼ cup coconut oil

3 teaspoons sweet almond oil

Directions:

Turn a saucepan onto medium low heat on your stove. Carefully scoop in the beeswax and stir until melted, then add in the shea butter and mango butter. Stir until these are melted as well.

Once you have a completely smooth blend, add in your coconut oil and almond oil, then the drops of essential oils.

Again, blend with a wooden spoon until completely smooth and carefully pour into airtight glass jars for storage.

When you are ready to use, simply scoop a small section out with your fingers (it will be firm) and let soften, then massage into your skin, and that's it!

Minty Mist

12 drops spearmint

10 drops wintergreen oil

1/8 cup shea butter

1/8 cup shredded mango butter

1/8 cup beeswax cubes

¼ cup coconut oil

3 teaspoons sweet almond oil

Directions:

Turn a saucepan onto medium low heat on your stove. Carefully scoop in the beeswax and stir until melted, then add in the shea butter and mango butter. Stir until these are melted as well.

Once you have a completely smooth blend, add in your coconut oil and almond oil, then the drops of essential oils.

Again, blend with a wooden spoon until completely smooth and carefully pour into airtight glass jars for storage.

When you are ready to use, simply scoop a small section out with your fingers (it will be firm) and let soften, then massage into your skin, and that's it!

Happy Summer Rays

10 drops orange

8 drops cinnamon

5 drops vanilla

1/8 cup shea butter

1/8 cup shredded mango butter

1/8 cup beeswax cubes

¼ cup coconut oil

3 teaspoons sweet almond oil

Directions:

Turn a saucepan onto medium low heat on your stove. Carefully scoop in the beeswax and stir until melted, then add in the shea butter and mango butter. Stir until these are melted as well.

Once you have a completely smooth blend, add in your coconut oil and almond oil, then the drops of essential oils.

Again, blend with a wooden spoon until completely smooth and carefully pour into airtight glass jars for storage.

When you are ready to use, simply scoop a small section out with your fingers (it will be firm) and let soften, then massage into your skin, and that's it!

A Night Out

10 drops popcorn aromatherapy oil

5 drops vanilla aromatherapy oil

1/8 cup shea butter

1/8 cup shredded mango butter

1/8 cup beeswax cubes

¼ cup coconut oil

3 teaspoons sweet almond oil

Directions:

Turn a saucepan onto medium low heat on your stove. Carefully scoop in the beeswax and stir until melted, then add in the shea butter and mango butter. Stir until these are melted as well.

Once you have a completely smooth blend, add in your coconut oil and almond oil, then the drops of essential oils.

Again, blend with a wooden spoon until completely smooth and carefully pour into airtight glass jars for storage.

When you are ready to use, simply scoop a small section out with your fingers (it will be firm) and let soften, then massage into your skin, and that's it!

The Carnival Hands

10 drops cotton candy aromatherapy oil

10 drops popcorn aromatherapy oil

5 drops cedar wood oil

1/8 cup shea butter

1/8 cup shredded mango butter

1/8 cup beeswax cubes

¼ cup coconut oil

3 teaspoons sweet almond oil

Directions:

Turn a saucepan onto medium low heat on your stove. Carefully scoop in the beeswax and stir until melted, then add in the shea butter and mango butter. Stir until these are melted as well.

Once you have a completely smooth blend, add in your coconut oil and almond oil, then the drops of essential oils.

Again, blend with a wooden spoon until completely smooth and carefully pour into airtight glass jars for storage.

When you are ready to use, simply scoop a small section out with your fingers (it will be firm) and let soften, then massage into your skin, and that's it!

Winter Summerland

10 drops peppermint

10 drops wintergreen

10 drops lavender

5 drops lemon

1/8 cup shea butter

1/8 cup shredded mango butter

1/8 cup beeswax cubes

¼ cup coconut oil

3 teaspoons sweet almond oil

Directions:

Turn a saucepan onto medium low heat on your stove. Carefully scoop in the beeswax and stir until melted, then add in the shea butter and mango butter. Stir until these are melted as well.

Once you have a completely smooth blend, add in your coconut oil and almond oil, then the drops of essential oils.

Again, blend with a wooden spoon until completely smooth and carefully pour into airtight glass jars for storage.

When you are ready to use, simply scoop a small section out with your fingers (it will be firm) and let soften, then massage into your skin, and that's it!

Happy Days

10 drops rose

10 drops grapefruit

10 drops cinnamon

10 drops peppermint

1/8 cup shea butter

1/8 cup shredded mango butter

1/8 cup beeswax cubes

¼ cup coconut oil

3 teaspoons sweet almond oil

Directions:

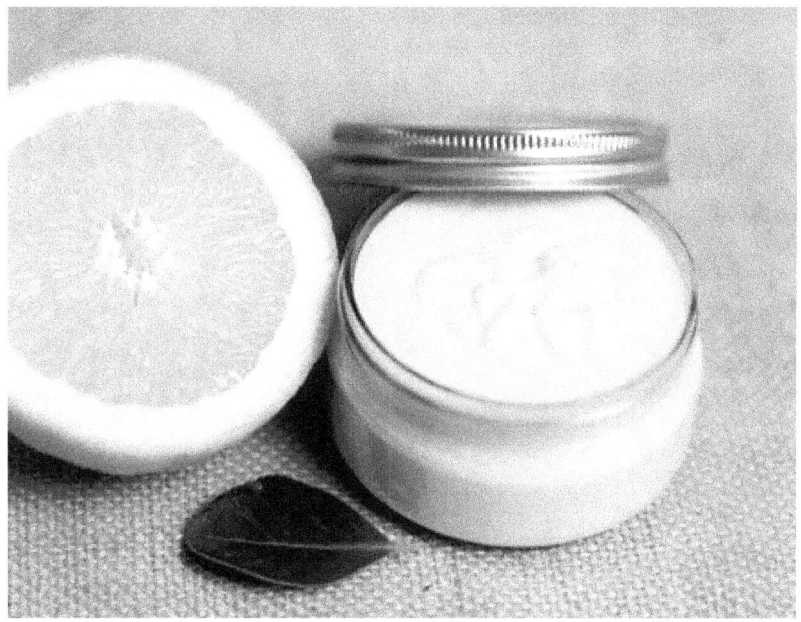

Turn a saucepan onto medium low heat on your stove. Carefully scoop in the beeswax and stir until melted, then add in the shea butter and mango butter. Stir until these are melted as well.

Once you have a completely smooth blend, add in your coconut oil and almond oil, then the drops of essential oils.

Again, blend with a wooden spoon until completely smooth and carefully pour into airtight glass jars for storage.

When you are ready to use, simply scoop a small section out with your fingers (it will be firm) and let soften, then massage into your skin, and that's it!

Perfection

12 drops eucalyptus

10 drops lemon

10 drops grapefruit

1/8 cup shea butter

1/8 cup shredded mango butter

1/8 cup beeswax cubes

¼ cup coconut oil

3 teaspoons sweet almond oil

Directions:

Turn a saucepan onto medium low heat on your stove. Carefully scoop in the beeswax and stir until melted, then add in the shea butter and mango butter. Stir until these are melted as well.

Once you have a completely smooth blend, add in your coconut oil and almond oil, then the drops of essential oils.

Again, blend with a wooden spoon until completely smooth and carefully pour into airtight glass jars for storage.

When you are ready to use, simply scoop a small section out with your fingers (it will be firm) and let soften, then massage into your skin, and that's it!

Chapter 5 – Lotion Bars

The Butter Bar

12 drops tea tree oil

15 drops peppermint

5 drops lilac oil

1/8 cup coconut oil

½ cup shredded beeswax

1/3 cup shea butter

Directions:

In a saucepan over medium low heat, melt the shea butter and the beeswax. Once melted, slowly add in the coconut oil, then the essential oils.

Pour into your molds, and let harden overnight.

Pop out of the molds, and store in a small glass jar, tin, or whatever you have on hand!

The Magic Moisturizer

10 drops ginger

10 drops cinnamon

5 drops patchouli

1/8 cup coconut oil

½ cup shredded beeswax

1/3 cup shea butter

Directions:

In a saucepan over medium low heat, melt the shea butter and the beeswax. Once melted, slowly add in the coconut oil, then the essential oils.

Pour into your molds, and let harden overnight.

Pop out of the molds, and store in a small glass jar, tin, or whatever you have on hand!

Firm But Fun

10 drops pine

10 drops cedar

10 drops peppermint

1/8 cup coconut oil

½ cup shredded beeswax

1/3 cup shea butter

Directions:

In a saucepan over medium low heat, melt the shea butter and the beeswax. Once melted, slowly add in the coconut oil, then the essential oils.

Pour into your molds, and let harden overnight.

Pop out of the molds, and store in a small glass jar, tin, or whatever you have on hand!

Lovey Scrubby

10 drops lavender

10 drops sunflower

10 drops hibiscus aromatherapy oil

1/8 cup coconut oil

½ cup shredded beeswax

1/3 cup shea butter

Directions:

In a saucepan over medium low heat, melt the shea butter and the beeswax. Once melted, slowly add in the coconut oil, then the essential oils.

Pour into your molds, and let harden overnight.

Pop out of the molds, and store in a small glass jar, tin, or whatever you have on hand!

The Twister Melt

10 drops caramel aromatherapy oil

10 drops green apple aromatherapy oil

1/8 cup coconut oil

½ cup shredded beeswax

1/3 cup shea butter

Directions:

In a saucepan over medium low heat, melt the shea butter and the beeswax. Once melted, slowly add in the coconut oil, then the essential oils.

Pour into your molds, and let harden overnight.

Pop out of the molds, and store in a small glass jar, tin, or whatever you have on hand!

Go Anywhere Silken Skein

10 drops basil

10 drops wintergreen

5 drops eucalyptus

1/8 cup coconut oil

½ cup shredded beeswax

1/3 cup shea butter

Directions:

In a saucepan over medium low heat, melt the shea butter and the beeswax. Once melted, slowly add in the coconut oil, then the essential oils.

Pour into your molds, and let harden overnight.

Pop out of the molds, and store in a small glass jar, tin, or whatever you have on hand!

The Perfect Purse Bar

10 drops hibiscus aromatherapy oil

10 drops lavender

5 drops lemon

1/8 cup coconut oil

½ cup shredded beeswax

1/3 cup shea butter

Directions:

In a saucepan over medium low heat, melt the shea butter and the beeswax. Once melted, slowly add in the coconut oil, then the essential oils.

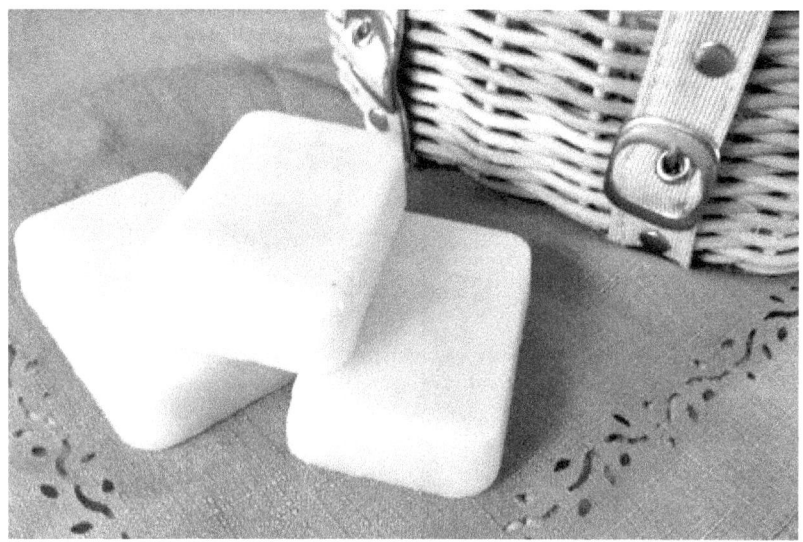

Pour into your molds, and let harden overnight.

Pop out of the molds, and store in a small glass jar, tin, or whatever you have on hand!

Moisture Madness

10 drops myrrh oil

10 drops frankincense

5 drops blood orange

1/8 cup coconut oil

½ cup shredded beeswax

1/3 cup shea butter

Directions:

In a saucepan over medium low heat, melt the shea butter and the beeswax. Once melted, slowly add in the coconut oil, then the essential oils.

Pour into your molds, and let harden overnight.

Pop out of the molds, and store in a small glass jar, tin, or whatever you have on hand!

Conclusion

There you have it, everything you need to know to make your own lotion, right at home!

I hope this book was able to show you that you can make your own lotions, and you can control exactly what goes into them, so you know without a doubt they are safe to have around every little one in your home.

I know you are going to fall in love with the process of making your own oils, and in no time at all you are going to want to make them for all occasions, or even no occasion at all.

When you make your own oils, you have the freedom to do what you want, when you want, without worrying about what you are putting on your skin, or if your little ones could get a hold of your lotion. Let this book bring your peace of mind as well as the freedom to do what you want with your lotions.

Go ahead and dive right in.

You deserve a little pampering.

FREE Bonus Reminder

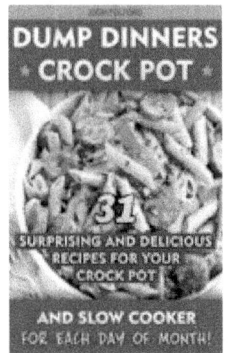

If you have not grabbed it yet, please go ahead and download your Free Ebook *"Dump Dinners Crock Pot: 31 Surprising And Delicious Recipes For Your Crock Pot And Slow Cooker For Each Day of Month!"*

Simply Click the Button Below

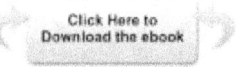

OR Go to This Page

http://easycookingideas.com/free

BONUS #2: More Free & Discounted Books & Products

Do you want to receive more Free/Discounted Books or Products?

We have a mailing list where we send out our new Books or Products when they go free or with a discount on Amazon. Click on the link below to sign up for Free & Discount Book & Product Promotions.

=> **Sign Up for Free & Discount Book & Products Promotions** <=

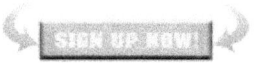

OR Go to this URL

http://zbit.ly/1WBb1Ek

www.ingramcontent.com/pod-product-compliance
Lightning Source LLC
Chambersburg PA
CBHW071135280526
45787CB00003B/1293